AYURVEDA COOKBOOK
FOR BEGINNERS

The Only guide You'll Need To
Balance Your Pitta Dosha For Joy,
Vitality, And General Well-Being

Alex kava

Copyright

No part of this publication may be reproduced, distributed, or transmitted in any form or by any means, including photocopying, recording, or other electronic or mechanical methods, without the prior written permission of the publisher, except in the case of brief quotations embodied in critical reviews and certain other noncommercial uses permitted by copyright law.

Table of Contents

Introduction

Once upon a time in a small town nestled between rolling hills and lush greenery, there lived a woman named Maya. Maya was an avid reader, and her quaint cottage was adorned with shelves filled with books on diverse subjects. However, one book had recently caught her eye—a simple yet intriguing title that read **"Ayurveda Cookbook for Beginners."**

Curiosity led Maya to delve into the pages of this book, and as she read about the ancient principles of Ayurveda, a newfound passion for mindful eating blossomed within her. The pages revealed the secrets of balancing the body and mind through nourishing foods and culinary practices. Each chapter seemed to unfold a world of flavors, textures, and health benefits.

Maya, being an adventurous soul, decided to embark on a culinary journey guided by the principles of Ayurveda. With the Ayurveda Cookbook as her compass, she explored the local markets, carefully selecting fresh and organic ingredients. She became attuned to the six tastes—sweet, sour, salty, bitter, pungent, and astringent—and discovered the art of combining them to create meals that were not only delicious but also tailored to her unique constitution.

In her cozy kitchen, Maya experimented with recipes that celebrated the seasons and the ever-changing tapestry of nature. She learned to appreciate the warming spices in winter and the cooling herbs in summer. Her culinary creations became a reflection of the harmony she sought to cultivate within herself.

As Maya prepared meals inspired by the Ayurveda Cookbook, her health and vitality began to flourish. She felt a renewed sense of energy, mental clarity, and a profound connection to the food she consumed. Friends and neighbors noticed the positive transformation in Maya and were eager to join her on this culinary adventure.

Maya's small cottage soon became a gathering place where she shared her newfound knowledge and the joy of Ayurvedic cooking. Together, they explored the vibrant world of spices, the healing properties of herbs, and the mindful art of savoring each bite. Laughter echoed in the air as they chopped vegetables, simmered aromatic stews, and embraced the principles of Ayurveda.

Word of Maya's culinary gatherings spread, reaching even the neighboring towns. The Ayurveda Cookbook for Beginners became a source of inspiration for many, guiding them toward a healthier and more harmonious way of life.

In the heart of this small town, Maya's cottage became a beacon of wellness, where the aroma of Ayurvedic spices mingled with the laughter of those who had discovered the joy of mindful eating. And so, Maya's story unfolded—a tale of transformation, shared meals, and the magic that happens when one embraces the wisdom of Ayurveda through the simple act of preparing a nourishing and balanced diet.

Chapter 1: Introduction to Ayurveda

Ayurveda, often referred to as the "science of life," is an ancient system of medicine that has its roots in the Indian subcontinent. The word "Ayurveda" is derived from the Sanskrit language, where "Ayur" means life, and "Veda" means knowledge or science. This holistic approach to healthcare has been practiced for thousands of years and continues to influence health and wellness practices around the world.

Historical Roots:

The origins of Ayurveda can be traced back to the Vedic period, around 5000 years ago. The knowledge and principles of Ayurveda were initially passed down orally through sacred texts, particularly the Vedas. Over time, these teachings were compiled into written texts, with the most significant being the Charaka Samhita and the Sushruta Samhita. These ancient texts form the foundation of Ayurvedic philosophy and provide detailed insights into the understanding of the human body, health, and disease.

Philosophy of Ayurveda:

Ayurveda operates on the fundamental principle that the human body is intricately connected to the universe and is composed of five basic elements: earth (prithvi), water (jal), fire (agni), air (vayu), and space (akasha). These elements combine to form three doshas—Vata, Pitta, and Kapha—which represent different combinations of the elements.

- **Vata:** Associated with the elements of air and space, Vata governs movement and is responsible for bodily functions like breathing, circulation, and elimination.

- **Pitta:** Aligned with the elements of fire and water, Pitta controls digestion, metabolism, and energy production within the body.

- **Kapha:** Comprising the elements of earth and water, Kapha is responsible for structure and lubrication, governing growth, stability, and immune function.

A balance of these doshas is crucial for maintaining good health, while an imbalance is believed to lead to illness. Ayurveda seeks to restore and maintain this balance through personalized lifestyle practices, dietary guidelines, herbal remedies, and various therapeutic techniques.

Holistic Approach:

One of the distinctive features of Ayurveda is its holistic approach to health. Rather than merely treating symptoms, Ayurvedic practitioners focus on identifying and addressing the root causes of imbalances in the body and mind. This approach considers the individual as a whole, taking into account physical, mental, and spiritual aspects.

Practices and Therapies:

Ayurveda offers a wide range of practices and therapies to promote health and well-being. These include:

- Dietary Guidelines: Ayurvedic nutrition emphasizes the importance of eating according to one's dosha to maintain balance.

- Herbal Medicine: The use of herbs and natural substances to address various health issues is a key aspect of Ayurvedic treatment.

- Yoga and Meditation: Physical postures (asanas) and meditation are integral to Ayurveda, promoting flexibility, strength, and mental clarity.

- Ayurvedic Massage and Therapies: Specialized massages and therapeutic techniques aim to balance the doshas and promote relaxation.

Modern Relevance:
While rooted in ancient traditions, Ayurveda continues to evolve and find relevance in the modern world. Its emphasis on preventive healthcare, personalized treatment plans, and holistic well-being has attracted attention globally. Ayurvedic principles are often integrated into complementary and alternative medicine practices,

offering individuals a holistic approach to health management.

Ayurveda stands as a timeless and comprehensive system of medicine, providing a holistic framework for understanding and cultivating a balanced and healthy life. Its enduring principles offer valuable insights into the intricate relationship between the individual and the cosmos, making it a source of wisdom that transcends cultural and geographical boundaries.

Understanding Ayurveda Principles

Ayurveda, often referred to as the "science of life," is an ancient system of medicine that traces its roots back to the Vedic period in India, around 5000 years ago. At its core, Ayurveda is a holistic approach to health and wellness, focusing on the interconnectedness of the body, mind, and spirit. The principles of Ayurveda provide a profound understanding of how the elements in nature influence our well-being and guide us toward a balanced and harmonious life.

The Five Elements and Three Doshas:
Ayurveda conceptualizes the universe and the human body in terms of five fundamental elements: earth (prithvi), water (jal), fire (agni), air (vayu), and space (akasha). These elements combine to form three dynamic forces or doshas: Vata, Pitta, and Kapha.

- Vata: Governed by the elements of air and space, Vata represents the force of movement. It is responsible for bodily functions such as breathing, circulation, and elimination.

- Pitta: Aligned with the elements of fire and water, Pitta embodies the force of transformation. It governs digestion, metabolism, and energy production in the body.

- Kapha: Comprising the elements of earth and water, Kapha represents the force of structure and stability. It governs growth, lubrication, and immune function.

The unique combination of these doshas in each individual determines their constitution, known as prakriti. Understanding one's prakriti is fundamental in Ayurveda as it guides personalized health recommendations and treatments.

Balancing the Doshas:

Ayurveda places a significant emphasis on maintaining a balance among the doshas to promote optimal health. Imbalances in these forces are believed to lead to various physical and mental ailments. Factors such as diet, lifestyle, seasons, and stress can influence the doshic balance.

- **Dietary Guidelines:** Ayurveda recommends dietary choices based on one's dosha to restore and maintain balance. For example, Vata individuals may benefit from warm, nourishing foods, while Pitta individuals may benefit from cooling and hydrating options.

- **Lifestyle Practices:** Daily routines, or dinacharya, are tailored to balance the doshas. This includes activities like oil massage, meditation, and exercise, aligning with the individual's constitution.

- **Herbal Remedies:** Ayurvedic medicine relies on a rich array of herbs and natural substances to address specific imbalances. These remedies aim to restore equilibrium and promote overall well-being.

Holistic Wellness:

Ayurveda perceives health as a dynamic state of balance that extends beyond the absence of disease. It recognizes the interconnectedness of physical, mental, and spiritual well-being, emphasizing the importance of nurturing a harmonious relationship with oneself and the environment.

- **Yoga and Meditation:** Physical postures (asanas) and meditation play a vital role in Ayurveda, promoting flexibility, strength, and mental clarity. These practices are integral to maintaining a balanced and centered state.

- **Mind-Body Connection:** Ayurveda acknowledges the influence of the mind on physical health and vice versa. Emotional well-being is considered crucial in preventing and managing diseases.

Modern Applications:

In the contemporary world, Ayurveda's principles are increasingly integrated into complementary and alternative medicine. Its focus on personalized care, preventive measures, and holistic well-being aligns with the growing interest in natural and holistic approaches to health.

Ayurveda offers a profound understanding of the principles that govern health and wellness. Its timeless wisdom provides a holistic framework for individuals to cultivate a balanced and harmonious life, fostering a deep connection between the self and the natural world.

The Three Doshas: Vata, Pitta, Kapha

Ayurveda, the ancient science of life, introduces a unique and fundamental concept that forms the cornerstone of its holistic approach to health: the three doshas. These doshas—Vata, Pitta, and Kapha—represent dynamic forces within the body, each governing specific physiological and psychological functions. Understanding the interplay of these doshas is key to achieving and maintaining balance in Ayurveda.

Vata: The Force of Movement

Vata is characterized by the elements of air and space, making it the force responsible for all movement in the body. It governs processes such as breathing, circulation, muscle contractions, and elimination. Individuals with a dominant Vata constitution tend to be creative, energetic, and quick-thinking. When Vata is in balance, it manifests as vitality, enthusiasm, and agility.

However, an excess of Vata can lead to conditions such as anxiety, insomnia, and digestive issues.

Balancing Vata:
- **Diet:** Warm, nourishing foods such as soups, stews, and cooked grains.
- **Lifestyle:** Establishing regular routines, practicing calming activities like meditation, and maintaining warmth in the environment.

Pitta: The Force of Transformation

Pitta is aligned with the elements of fire and water, representing the force responsible for transformation and metabolic processes. It governs digestion, absorption, and the body's thermal regulation. Pitta-dominant individuals are often characterized by their sharp intellect, strong leadership qualities, and a warm demeanor. In balance, Pitta promotes a healthy appetite, sharp mental focus, and effective digestion. Imbalances can lead to issues like inflammation, acidity, and irritability.

Balancing Pitta:

- **Diet:** Cooling and hydrating foods, such as leafy greens, cucumber, and coconut.

- **Lifestyle:** Engaging in calming activities, avoiding excessive heat, and ensuring a balanced work-play routine.

Kapha: The Force of Structure and Stability

Kapha, governed by the elements of earth and water, embodies the force of structure and stability. It is responsible for maintaining the body's form, providing lubrication, and supporting the immune system. Individuals with a predominant Kapha constitution are often steady, nurturing, and have a robust physique. A balanced Kapha fosters strength, endurance, and emotional calm. However, an excess can lead to conditions like lethargy, weight gain, and congestion.

Balancing Kapha:

- **Diet:** Light and warming foods, incorporating spices, and reducing heavy or sweet foods.

- Lifestyle: Regular exercise, engaging in stimulating activities, and maintaining a warm and dry environment.

Prakriti and Vikriti: Understanding Individual Constitution and Imbalance

In Ayurveda, every individual has a unique combination of the three doshas known as prakriti, determined at the time of conception. Understanding one's prakriti provides insights into inherent strengths and susceptibilities. Additionally, Ayurveda recognizes vikriti, the current state of doshic balance influenced by factors like diet, lifestyle, and environmental conditions.

Balancing Doshas for Overall Well-being:
- Self-awareness: Regularly assessing one's state of well-being and adjusting lifestyle practices accordingly.
- Holistic Approach: Incorporating Ayurvedic practices such as yoga, meditation, and herbal remedies to maintain doshic equilibrium.

The three doshas—Vata, Pitta, and Kapha—constitute the foundational framework of Ayurveda. This ancient wisdom recognizes the dynamic and ever-changing nature of the human body, providing personalized guidelines to foster balance, harmony, and optimal health in individuals.

Importance of Balancing Pitta for Well-Being

In the ancient science of Ayurveda, the concept of the three doshas—Vata, Pitta, and Kapha—plays a crucial role in understanding individual constitutions and maintaining overall well-being. Among these doshas, Pitta, associated with the elements of fire and water, holds a central place in the balance of bodily functions. Balancing Pitta is considered essential in Ayurveda for promoting physical health, emotional harmony, and mental clarity.

Pitta: The Force of Transformation

Pitta is responsible for the transformative processes within the body, encompassing digestion, absorption, and assimilation of nutrients. It governs metabolism, body temperature, and the production of enzymes and hormones. Individuals with a predominant Pitta constitution tend to possess qualities such as intensity, focus, and a warm disposition. When Pitta is in balance, it contributes to a strong digestive system, clear complexion, and a sharp intellect.

Importance of Balancing Pitta:

1. Digestive Health:

- **Balanced Pitta:** Supports efficient digestion and absorption of nutrients, preventing issues like indigestion, heartburn, and inflammation.

- **Imbalanced Pitta:** Can lead to excessive acidity, ulcers, and inflammatory conditions in the digestive tract.

2. Emotional Equilibrium:

- **Balanced Pitta:** Promotes emotional stability, confidence, and a positive outlook on life.

- **Imbalanced Pitta:** May manifest as irritability, anger, frustration, and heightened stress levels.

3. Skin Health:

- **Balanced Pitta:** Contributes to a healthy and radiant complexion.

- **Imbalanced Pitta:** Can result in skin conditions such as acne, rashes, or sensitivity.

4. Temperature Regulation:

- **Balanced Pitta:** Maintains a regulated body temperature.

- **Imbalanced Pitta:** May lead to heat-related issues, excessive sweating, and sensitivity to hot weather.

5. Hormonal Harmony:

- **Balanced Pitta:** Supports the proper production and balance of hormones.

- **Imbalanced Pitta:** Can disrupt hormonal equilibrium, potentially leading to menstrual irregularities, hot flashes, or mood swings.

Balancing Pitta: Ayurvedic Recommendations:

1. Dietary Guidelines:

- Incorporate cooling foods such as cucumbers, mint, and coconut.

- Reduce spicy, oily, and acidic foods that can aggravate Pitta.

2. Lifestyle Practices:

- Engage in calming activities such as meditation, deep breathing, and gentle yoga.

- Establish a balanced work-play routine to manage stress.

3. Herbal Remedies:

- Use herbs with cooling properties, such as aloe vera, coriander, and fennel.

- Ayurvedic formulations tailored to balance Pitta may include specific herbs to soothe the digestive system and calm the mind.

4. Mindful Sun Exposure:

- Be mindful of exposure to the sun, as excessive heat can exacerbate Pitta imbalances.

- Seek shade during peak sunlight hours and stay hydrated.

In Ayurveda, the significance of balancing Pitta cannot be overstated. Achieving and maintaining harmony within the Pitta dosha contributes not only to physical health but also to emotional and mental well-being. By adopting Ayurvedic principles tailored to balance Pitta, individuals can cultivate a state of equilibrium that supports their overall health and vitality.

Chapter 2: Discovering Your Pitta Dosha

Ayurveda, the ancient science of holistic health, places great emphasis on understanding individual constitutions, known as doshas, to tailor lifestyle choices and promote well-being. Among the three doshas—Vata, Pitta, and Kapha—Pitta is associated with the elements of fire and water, governing transformation and metabolic processes. Discovering your Pitta dosha involves recognizing both your inherent tendencies, known as prakriti, and your current state of doshic balance, known as vikriti. Here's a guide to help you explore and understand your Pitta dosha:

1. Recognizing Pitta Characteristics:
  - **Physical Traits:** Individuals with a predominant Pitta dosha often have a medium build, a strong metabolism, and a tendency to easily gain or lose weight.

- **Skin Type:** Pitta-dominant individuals typically have sensitive, fair, and warm-toned skin that may be prone to rashes or inflammations.

- **Hair:** Pitta-influenced hair is often fine and may exhibit premature graying or thinning.

2. Identifying Pitta Mental and Emotional Traits:

- **Mental Acuity:** Pitta individuals are known for their sharp intellect, strong analytical skills, and a keen ability to focus on tasks.

- **Emotional Characteristics:** While Pitta fosters leadership qualities and a natural drive, imbalances may manifest as irritability, impatience, or a tendency towards perfectionism.

3. Assessing Digestive Patterns:

- **Appetite:** Pitta individuals typically have a strong appetite and efficient digestion.

- **Tolerance to Heat:** Pitta is associated with the element of fire, so a Pitta-dominant person may have a moderate tolerance for heat and may be more prone to overheating.

4. Understanding Your Reaction to Stress:

- **Stress Response:** Pitta individuals may respond to stress with intensity and may experience physical symptoms such as digestive discomfort, headaches, or skin issues.

- **Need for Relaxation:** Balancing Pitta requires intentional efforts to engage in calming activities, as stress can exacerbate Pitta imbalances.

5. Determining Prakriti and Vikriti:

- **Prakriti:** Your inherent constitution, or prakriti, is determined at the time of conception and represents your unique combination of the three doshas. Take an Ayurvedic dosha quiz or consult with an Ayurvedic practitioner to identify your prakriti.

- **Vikriti:** Your current state of doshic balance, or vikriti, can be influenced by lifestyle, diet, and environmental factors. Observing changes in your physical and mental well-being can provide insights into your current doshic state.

6. Ayurvedic Consultation:

- **Professional Guidance:** For a comprehensive understanding of your Pitta dosha, consider consulting with an Ayurvedic practitioner. They can assess your prakriti, vikriti, and provide personalized recommendations to balance Pitta through dietary choices, lifestyle adjustments, and herbal remedies.

7. Lifestyle Adjustments to Balance Pitta:

- **Diet:** Emphasize cooling and hydrating foods such as leafy greens, cucumbers, and sweet fruits. Minimize spicy, oily, and acidic foods.

- **Lifestyle Practices:** Engage in calming activities like meditation, gentle yoga, and spending time in nature. Maintain a balanced work-play routine.

- **Herbal Support:** Explore Ayurvedic herbs with cooling properties, such as aloe vera, coriander, and shatavari.

Discovering your Pitta dosha is a journey of self-awareness that allows you to align your lifestyle with your unique constitution. By embracing Ayurvedic principles and making intentional choices, you can foster balance, vitality, and well-being in your life.

Pitta Characteristics and Traits

In Ayurveda, the ancient system of holistic medicine, understanding your dosha is key to personalized well-being. Among the three doshas—Vata, Pitta, and Kapha—Pitta, governed by the elements of fire and water, holds distinctive characteristics that influence both physical and mental attributes. Recognizing these Pitta traits is crucial in tailoring lifestyle choices to maintain balance and promote optimal health.

1. Physical Traits:

  - **Medium Build:** Pitta-dominant individuals often have a medium build with well-defined musculature.
  - **Sharp Features:** Facial features tend to be sharp and well-defined, reflecting the intensity associated with Pitta.
  - **Warm Complexion:** The skin tends to be fair, warm-toned, and may exhibit a tendency towards sensitivity.

2. Metabolism and Digestion:

- **Strong Metabolism:** Pitta is associated with the transformative power of fire, contributing to a robust and efficient metabolism.

- **Acidic Stomach:** Pitta individuals may have a tendency towards acidity and may benefit from a balanced diet to soothe the digestive system.

3. Hair and Eyes:

- **Fine Hair:** Pitta-influenced hair is often fine and silky in texture.

- **Penetrating Eyes:** The eyes are typically sharp, penetrating, and may display intensity.

4. Mental Acuity:

- **Sharp Intellect:** Pitta individuals are known for their sharp intellect, analytical skills, and a natural ability to focus.

- **Leadership Qualities:** There is a natural inclination towards leadership, assertiveness, and a drive to achieve goals.

5. Emotions and Personality Traits:

- **Passionate Nature:** Pitta individuals exhibit a passionate and enthusiastic approach to life.

- **Intensity:** While they are driven and focused, imbalances can lead to heightened emotions such as irritability, impatience, or frustration.

6. Response to Stress:

- **Stressful Situations:** Pitta individuals may respond to stress with intensity, potentially experiencing physical symptoms like headaches or digestive discomfort.

- **Need for Relaxation:** Balancing Pitta requires intentional efforts to engage in calming activities, as stress can exacerbate Pitta imbalances.

7. Appetite and Food Preferences:

- **Strong Appetite:** Pitta-dominant individuals typically have a strong and efficient digestive system.

- **Favoring Cooling Foods:** They may have a natural preference for cooling foods such as salads, fruits, and mint-infused beverages.

8. Tolerance to Heat:

- Moderate Heat Tolerance: Pitta is associated with the fire element, and individuals with a dominant Pitta dosha may have a moderate tolerance for heat.

9. Sleep Patterns:

- Quality Sleep: When balanced, Pitta individuals enjoy restful and refreshing sleep.

- Potential for Sleep Disturbances: Imbalances may lead to difficulty falling asleep, vivid dreams, or waking up feeling overheated.

10. Communication Style:

- Clear and Direct: Pitta individuals tend to communicate in a clear, direct, and assertive manner.

- Articulate Expression: They often express themselves with precision and articulate their thoughts effectively.

Understanding these Pitta characteristics provides a foundation for discovering your dosha and personalizing your lifestyle choices. By embracing Ayurvedic principles and making adjustments tailored to your unique constitution, you can foster balance, vitality, and well-being in your life. If you're curious about your dosha composition, consider taking an Ayurvedic dosha quiz or consulting with an Ayurvedic practitioner for personalized insights.

Dosha Quiz: Identifying Your Dominant Dosha

Embarking on the journey of self-discovery in Ayurveda involves understanding your unique constitution, or dosha, which influences your physical, mental, and emotional well-being. One effective way to identify your dominant dosha is by taking a dosha quiz. This self-assessment tool helps individuals gain insights into their inherent tendencies, guiding them towards a more personalized approach to health and lifestyle choices. Below are key aspects to consider when taking a dosha quiz to identify your dominant dosha, with a focus on the Pitta dosha.

1. Dosha Quiz Structure:

- Dosha quizzes typically comprise a series of questions covering various aspects of your physical, mental, and emotional states.

- Questions may explore your body type, digestion, sleep patterns, mental attributes, and responses to stress.

2. Physical Attributes:

- Questions may assess your body build, skin type, hair texture, and other physical characteristics associated with each dosha.

- Pitta-dominant individuals may resonate with questions related to a medium build, warm skin tone, and fine hair.

3. Digestive Patterns:

- Queries about your appetite, digestion, and preferences for certain foods help determine your digestive tendencies.

- A strong appetite, efficient digestion, and a preference for cooling foods may align with Pitta characteristics.

4. Mental and Emotional Traits:

- Questions may delve into your mental acuity, emotional responses, and overall temperament.

- A sharp intellect, leadership qualities, and a tendency towards intensity may indicate a dominant Pitta dosha.

5. Stress Response:

- The quiz may explore how you respond to stress, examining both emotional and physical reactions.

- Pitta individuals may exhibit heightened emotions and may experience symptoms such as headaches or digestive discomfort under stress.

6. Sleep Patterns:

- Questions related to your sleep habits, quality, and any disturbances can provide insights into your doshic balance.

- Pitta-dominant individuals typically enjoy restful sleep when balanced but may experience sleep disturbances when imbalanced.

7. Communication Style:

- Queries about your communication preferences, assertiveness, and clarity of expression may be included.

- A direct, clear, and assertive communication style aligns with Pitta characteristics.

8. Lifestyle Preferences:

- The dosha quiz may inquire about your preferences for daily routines, exercise, and environmental factors.

- Pitta individuals may resonate with choices that incorporate cooling activities, moderate exercise, and a balanced work-play routine.

9. Seasonal Preferences:

- Questions about how you feel in different seasons can provide clues about your doshic tendencies.

- Pitta individuals may enjoy cooler seasons and may need to take precautions to balance the heat during warmer months.

10. Dosha Scoring:

- After completing the quiz, the scoring system will identify the dosha or doshas that are most dominant in your constitution.

- A higher score in Pitta-related questions suggests a dominant Pitta dosha.

Dosha Quiz Considerations:

- It's important to note that dosha quizzes provide general insights and are not definitive diagnostic tools.

- Dosha imbalances can change over time, influenced by factors such as diet, lifestyle, and environment.

Taking a dosha quiz is a valuable first step in discovering your dominant dosha, particularly if you resonate with the Pitta characteristics. However, for a more accurate and personalized assessment, consider consulting with an Ayurvedic practitioner who can provide tailored insights and recommendations based on a comprehensive understanding of your unique constitution.

Personalized Ayurvedic Assessment

While dosha quizzes offer a convenient introduction to Ayurveda and can provide valuable insights into your dominant dosha, a personalized Ayurvedic assessment takes the exploration of your constitution to a deeper and more comprehensive level. Conducted by trained Ayurvedic practitioners, this assessment involves a thorough examination of various aspects of your physical, mental, and emotional states to offer targeted recommendations for achieving and maintaining doshic balance, particularly focusing on the Pitta dosha.

1. In-Depth Consultation:

- An Ayurvedic assessment typically begins with a detailed consultation with an experienced practitioner.

- During this session, the practitioner explores various facets of your life, including your medical history, daily routines, dietary habits, and emotional well-being.

2. Pulse Diagnosis (Nadi Pariksha):

- One of the unique aspects of Ayurvedic assessment is pulse diagnosis, known as Nadi Pariksha.

- Practitioners skilled in Nadi Pariksha can detect subtle imbalances in the doshas by analyzing the pulse at different points on the wrist.

3. Tongue Examination:

- The examination of the tongue can reveal information about the state of digestion and the presence of any potential imbalances.

- Pitta imbalances may be indicated by a yellowish or reddish discoloration of the tongue.

4. Observation of Physical Characteristics:

- The practitioner observes physical traits such as body build, skin texture, hair type, and facial features.

- Pitta characteristics, such as a medium build, warm complexion, and fine hair, are considered in the assessment.

5. Assessment of Digestive Patterns:

- Your digestive tendencies, including appetite, metabolism, and reactions to certain foods, are carefully assessed.

- Pitta-dominant individuals may be advised on dietary choices to pacify excess heat and acidity.

6. Evaluation of Mental and Emotional Well-being:

- The practitioner explores your mental acuity, emotional responses, and overall temperament.

- Pitta individuals may receive recommendations to manage stress and prevent emotional imbalances.

7. Lifestyle Analysis:

- Your daily routines, sleep patterns, and environmental factors are analyzed to identify areas for improvement.

- Pitta individuals may be guided to adopt cooling practices, maintain a balanced work-play routine, and manage exposure to heat.

8. Customized Recommendations:

- Based on the findings of the assessment, the Ayurvedic practitioner provides personalized recommendations tailored to your unique constitution.

- Specific dietary guidelines, lifestyle adjustments, herbal remedies, and therapeutic practices may be suggested to balance Pitta.

9. Follow-Up Sessions:

- Ayurvedic assessments often include follow-up sessions to monitor progress and make further adjustments to the recommendations.

- Regular check-ins with the practitioner allow for ongoing support and refinement of your Ayurvedic plan.

10. Integration of Ayurvedic Practices:

- The personalized assessment aims to integrate Ayurvedic practices seamlessly into your daily life.

- Practices such as specific yoga asanas, meditation techniques, and self-care rituals may be recommended to enhance well-being.

A personalized Ayurvedic assessment offers a holistic and nuanced understanding of your unique constitution and imbalances. It empowers you with targeted strategies to balance your Pitta dosha, fostering optimal health and vitality. Consider consulting with a qualified Ayurvedic practitioner for a comprehensive assessment that aligns with your individual needs and goals.

Chapter 3: Pitta Pacifying Foods

In Ayurveda, maintaining balance among the doshas—Vata, Pitta, and Kapha—is essential for overall well-being. For individuals with a predominant Pitta dosha, characterized by the elements of fire and water, adopting a diet that pacifies excess heat and promotes cooling is crucial. Pitta-pacifying foods play a significant role in harmonizing this dosha, supporting digestion, and promoting emotional equilibrium. Here is a guide to the key characteristics and examples of Pitta pacifying foods:

1. Cooling Fruits:

 - **Sweet Fruits:** Opt for sweet and juicy fruits like sweet melons, grapes, mangoes, and ripe pears.

 - **Berries:** Blueberries, strawberries, and raspberries provide antioxidant benefits and are cooling in nature.

2. Sweet and Bitter Vegetables:

- **Leafy Greens:** Embrace cooling greens such as spinach, kale, and Swiss chard.

- **Bitter Vegetables:** Include bitter vegetables like bitter gourd, dandelion greens, and Brussels sprouts to balance Pitta.

3. Grains:

- **Basmati Rice:** Choose basmati rice as a cooling and easily digestible option.

- **Quinoa:** This grain is not only high in protein but also has a cooling effect on the body.

4. Dairy and Alternatives:

- **Milk:** Cow's milk, when consumed in moderation, has a cooling effect. Consider coconut or almond milk as dairy alternatives.

- **Ghee:** Clarified butter is beneficial in moderation for Pitta individuals.

5. Cooling Spices:

- **Coriander:** Both the seeds and fresh leaves (cilantro) are cooling and can be used in various dishes.

- Fennel: Fennel seeds can be included in meals or consumed as a digestive tea.

6. Sweeteners:

- Sweeteners: Opt for natural sweeteners like honey, maple syrup, or stevia in moderation.

- Coconut Sugar: A sweetener with a lower glycemic index, coconut sugar can be a Pitta-friendly alternative.

7. Nuts and Seeds:

- Coconut: Fresh coconut and coconut products have cooling properties.

- Sunflower Seeds: Sunflower seeds are a nutritious and cooling snack option.

8. Cooling Beverages:

- Mint Tea: A refreshing and cooling option, mint tea can be enjoyed hot or cold.

- Cucumber Juice: Cucumber is hydrating and cooling, making it an excellent choice for Pitta individuals.

9. Sweet and Cooling Desserts:

- **Fruit Sorbet:** Homemade sorbets made from Pitta-pacifying fruits can satisfy sweet cravings.

- **Rice Pudding:** A cooling and soothing dessert made with basmati rice and milk.

10. Moderation is Key:

- While emphasizing cooling foods, Pitta individuals should also focus on moderation in their diet to prevent excess.

Avoid or Limit:

- **Spicy Foods:** Minimize or avoid overly spicy foods that can aggravate Pitta.

- **Sour Foods:** Reduce intake of sour foods, such as citrus fruits and vinegar.

- **Excessive Salt:** High salt intake can contribute to Pitta imbalances; opt for moderate salt levels.

Balancing with Mindful Eating:

- **Meal Timing:** Regular meal times and avoiding skipping meals can help maintain digestive balance.

- **Mindful Eating:** Eating in a calm and focused manner, avoiding rushed meals, contributes to balanced digestion.

Incorporating Pitta pacifying foods into your diet can help manage excess heat, support digestion, and foster emotional balance. It's essential to listen to your body and make dietary choices that align with your unique constitution. Consulting with an Ayurvedic practitioner for personalized guidance can provide further insights into optimizing your diet and lifestyle for Pitta balance.

Cooling Foods to Balance Pitta

In Ayurveda, the Pitta dosha, associated with the elements of fire and water, governs metabolic processes and transformation in the body. When Pitta becomes imbalanced, individuals may experience symptoms such as acidity, inflammation, and heightened emotional intensity. Adopting a diet rich in cooling, Pitta-pacifying foods is a key strategy to restore balance, support digestion, and promote overall well-being. Here is a guide to cooling foods that can help balance Pitta dosha:

1. Sweet and Juicy Fruits:

- **Melons:** Watermelon, cantaloupe, and honeydew are hydrating and have a cooling effect.

- **Berries:** Blueberries, strawberries, and raspberries are antioxidant-rich and contribute to a balanced Pitta.

2. Leafy Greens:

- **Spinach:** High in vitamins and minerals, spinach is cooling and can be incorporated into salads or cooked dishes.

- **Kale:** A nutrient-dense green that can be included in smoothies or lightly sautéed.

3. Cucumber:

- **Cucumber:** With its high water content, cucumber is incredibly hydrating and cooling.

- **Cucumber Raita:** A traditional Indian dish made with yogurt, cucumber, and cooling spices.

4. Zucchini and Summer Squash:

- **Zucchini:** Light and easily digestible, zucchini is a versatile vegetable that can be included in various dishes.

- **Summer Squash:** Delicate and mild, summer squash can be a soothing addition to meals.

5. Coconut:

- **Coconut:** Both the flesh and water of coconuts have a cooling effect. Coconut milk is a suitable dairy alternative.

- **Coconut Water:** Refreshing and hydrating, coconut water is an excellent choice for Pitta individuals.

6. Mint:

- **Fresh Mint:** Mint leaves can be used in salads, teas, or infused water for a cooling flavor.

- **Mint Chutney:** A flavorful condiment made with fresh mint, cilantro, and cooling spices.

7. Cilantro:

- **Cilantro (Coriander):** Cilantro has cooling properties and can be added to salads, salsas, or garnishes.

- **Coriander Tea:** Coriander seeds can be used to make a soothing tea to balance Pitta.

8. Fennel:

- **Fennel:** Fennel seeds can be chewed after meals to aid digestion and provide a cooling effect.
- **Roasted Fennel:** A delightful side dish, roasted fennel adds a unique flavor to meals.

9. Basmati Rice:

- **Basmati Rice:** A light and aromatic rice variety that is easy to digest and has a cooling influence.
- **Quinoa:** An alternative grain that is both nutritious and cooling for Pitta.

10. Dairy in Moderation:

- **Milk:** Cow's milk, in moderation, can have a cooling effect. Consider dairy alternatives like coconut or almond milk.
- **Ghee:** Clarified butter, in small amounts, is well-tolerated and can be used for cooking.

11. Sweeteners in Moderation:

- **Honey:** Raw, unpasteurized honey is a sweetener with cooling properties when consumed in moderation.

- **Coconut Sugar:** A Pitta-friendly alternative with a lower glycemic index.

12. Aloe Vera:

- **Aloe Vera:** Aloe vera juice can be consumed in small quantities to cool and soothe the digestive system.

Tips for Pitta-Pacifying Eating:

- **Meal Timing:** Stick to regular meal times to support balanced digestion.

- **Mindful Eating:** Enjoy meals in a calm environment, savoring each bite mindfully.

Balancing Pitta dosha with cooling foods is not just about what you eat but also how you eat. By incorporating these Pitta-pacifying foods into your diet and adopting mindful eating practices, you can support your body's natural ability to stay cool, calm, and in balance. If you have specific health concerns or seek personalized guidance, consulting with an Ayurvedic practitioner can provide tailored recommendations for your unique constitution.

Ayurvedic Superfoods for Pitta Dosha

Ayurveda, the ancient system of holistic healing, emphasizes the importance of diet in maintaining balance among the doshas. For individuals with a predominant Pitta dosha, incorporating Ayurvedic superfoods that possess cooling and balancing properties is key to supporting overall well-being. These superfoods not only nourish the body but also help pacify excess heat and inflammation associated with Pitta dosha. Here's a guide to Ayurvedic superfoods for Pitta dosha:

1. Amalaki (Indian Gooseberry):
   - **Benefits:** Amalaki is a potent rejuvenating fruit with high vitamin C content. It supports digestion, promotes healthy skin, and has a cooling effect.

- **Usage:** Fresh amalaki, amalaki powder, or amalaki supplements can be incorporated into your diet.

2. Shatavari:

- **Benefits:** Shatavari is a nourishing herb known for its cooling properties. It supports reproductive health, balances hormones, and soothes the digestive system.

- **Usage:** Shatavari powder or capsules can be taken as a supplement, or the root can be used in teas and infusions.

3. Aloe Vera:

- **Benefits:** Aloe vera has cooling and soothing properties, making it beneficial for digestive health. It helps alleviate inflammation and supports skin health.

- **Usage:** Fresh aloe vera gel can be added to smoothies, consumed as a juice, or applied topically.

4. Guduchi (Tinospora Cordifolia):

- **Benefits:** Guduchi is a powerful herb known for its immune-boosting and anti-inflammatory properties. It helps cool the body and supports detoxification.

- **Usage:** Guduchi supplements, powders, or decoctions can be included in your daily routine.

5. Coconut:

- **Benefits:** Coconut, in various forms, has cooling and hydrating effects. It supports digestion, nourishes the skin, and provides essential fatty acids.

- **Usage:** Fresh coconut, coconut water, coconut milk, and coconut oil can be incorporated into cooking and beverages.

6. Turmeric:

- **Benefits:** Turmeric possesses anti-inflammatory properties and supports the liver. It can help balance Pitta without overheating the body.

- **Usage:** Include turmeric in curries, soups, or golden milk. Turmeric supplements are also available.

7. Ghee (Clarified Butter):

- **Benefits:** Ghee is a Pitta-friendly source of healthy fats that supports digestion, enhances nutrient absorption, and has a cooling effect.

- **Usage:** Use ghee in cooking or add a small amount to dishes for flavor.

8. Coriander:

- **Benefits:** Coriander is cooling and aids digestion. Both the seeds and fresh leaves (cilantro) can be used to balance Pitta.

- **Usage:** Coriander seeds in teas, coriander powder in cooking, and fresh cilantro in salads and garnishes.

9. Fennel:

- **Benefits:** Fennel has cooling and digestive properties. It helps alleviate bloating and supports overall digestive health.

- **Usage:** Fennel seeds can be chewed after meals or used in teas. Fresh fennel can be added to salads.

10. Mung Beans:

- **Benefits:** Mung beans are easy to digest and have a cooling effect. They provide a good source of protein without overly stimulating Pitta.

- **Usage:** Include mung beans in soups, stews, or as a base for salads.

11. Sandalwood:

- **Benefits:** Sandalwood has a cooling and calming effect. It is traditionally used to cool the skin and balance Pitta.

- **Usage:** Sandalwood paste or oil can be applied topically. Sandalwood supplements are also available.

12. Cardamom:

- **Benefits:** Cardamom is a cooling spice that supports digestion and helps balance Pitta without aggravating heat.

- **Usage:** Add cardamom to teas, desserts, or sprinkle it on foods.

Incorporating Ayurvedic superfoods for Pitta dosha into your diet can contribute to maintaining balance, supporting digestive health, and promoting overall vitality. As with any dietary changes, it's advisable to consult with an Ayurvedic practitioner for personalized recommendations based on your unique constitution and health goals.

Creating a Pitta–Friendly Kitchen

In Ayurveda, the kitchen is considered the heart of the home, and the choices made in this space have a profound impact on one's well-being. For individuals with a predominant Pitta dosha, creating a Pitta-friendly kitchen involves thoughtful selection of ingredients, cooking methods, and kitchen practices that help maintain balance and support digestive health. Here's a guide to transforming your kitchen into a Pitta-pacifying space:

1. Choose Cooling Ingredients:
   - **Fruits:** Stock your kitchen with cooling fruits such as sweet melons, berries, and ripe pears.
   - **Vegetables:** Embrace leafy greens, cucumbers, zucchini, and bitter vegetables like bitter gourd.

- **Herbs:** Incorporate cooling herbs like mint, cilantro (coriander), and fennel into your recipes.

2. Opt for Pitta-Pacifying Grains:

- **Basmati Rice:** Choose basmati rice for its cooling and easily digestible qualities.
- **Quinoa:** A nutritious alternative that complements a Pitta-balancing diet.

3. Include Pitta-Friendly Proteins:

- **Mung Beans:** Easily digestible and cooling, mung beans are an excellent protein source.
- **Dairy in Moderation:** Include moderate amounts of cooling dairy like milk, ghee, and yogurt.

4. Incorporate Pitta-Balancing Spices:

- **Coriander:** Use coriander in your spice blends and cooking. Both the seeds and fresh leaves (cilantro) are cooling.
- **Cardamom:** Add cardamom to teas, desserts, and savory dishes for its cooling effect.

5. Choose Pitta-Soothing Oils:

- **Coconut Oil:** A cooling oil that can be used for cooking and baking.

- **Ghee:** Clarified butter, in moderation, is suitable for Pitta dosha.

6. Embrace Pitta-Friendly Cooking Methods:

- **Steaming:** Opt for steaming to retain the natural moisture and nutrients in foods.

- **Boiling:** Boil vegetables, grains, and legumes to preserve their cooling properties.

- **Raw Preparations:** Include raw salads and snacks for a refreshing and cooling touch.

7. Mindful Meal Timing:

- **Regular Meal Times:** Establish regular meal times to support a balanced digestive fire.

- **Avoid Skipping Meals:** Skipping meals can provoke Pitta; ensure you eat at consistent intervals.

8. Pitta-Pacifying Beverages:

- **Cooling Teas:** Enjoy herbal teas like mint, coriander, or fennel to stay hydrated and cool.

- **Coconut Water:** A hydrating and refreshing beverage for Pitta individuals.

9. Create a Calming Atmosphere:**
- **Soft Colors:** Opt for soft, calming colors in your kitchen, such as shades of blue and green.
- **Dim Lighting:** Soft, dim lighting creates a soothing ambiance.

10. Organize with Intention:
- **Keep it Clean:** A clutter-free kitchen promotes a calm environment.
- **Label Ingredients:** Clearly label spices and ingredients for easy access and organization.

11. Mindful Storage of Leftovers:
- **Avoid Overnight Refrigeration:** Whenever possible, consume freshly prepared meals.
- **Store in Glass Containers:** If storing leftovers, use glass containers to avoid leaching from plastic.

12. Seasonal Awareness:

- **Incorporate Seasonal Foods:** Adjust your kitchen choices based on seasonal produce to stay in harmony with nature.

- **Avoid Heating Foods in Summer:** During hot seasons, reduce the consumption of heating foods like spicy curries.

13. Cooking with Love and Intention:

- **Infuse Love into Meals:** Prepare meals with love and positive intentions for nourishing energy.

- **Practice Mindful Cooking:** Be present in the moment while preparing food, allowing the process to be a meditative experience.

By incorporating these Pitta-pacifying elements into your kitchen, you create a space that aligns with Ayurvedic principles, fostering balance, harmony, and well-being. For personalized guidance tailored to your unique constitution and health goals, consider consulting with an Ayurvedic practitioner who can provide insights into creating a kitchen environment that supports your Pitta dosha.

Chapter 4: Joyful Pitta Recipes

Cooking with joy and creativity is not only a culinary art but also an expression of self-care. For individuals with a predominant Pitta dosha, choosing recipes that incorporate cooling and balancing ingredients is key to maintaining harmony and well-being. Here are some joyful Pitta recipes that not only cater to the specific needs of Pitta dosha but also bring joy and satisfaction to the dining experience:

1. Cooling Cucumber Mint Salad:
  - Ingredients:
    - Cucumbers, thinly sliced
    - Fresh mint leaves, chopped
    - Feta cheese, crumbled (optional)
    - Olive oil
    - Lemon juice
    - Salt and pepper to taste
  - Instructions:

- Toss sliced cucumbers, chopped mint, and crumbled feta (if using) in a bowl.

- Drizzle with olive oil and fresh lemon juice.

- Season with salt and pepper to taste. Refrigerate before serving for extra coolness.

2. Quinoa and Vegetable Buddha Bowl:

- Ingredients:

- Cooked quinoa
- Steamed broccoli florets
- Sliced bell peppers (preferably red or yellow)
- Shredded carrots
- Avocado slices
- Tahini dressing

- Instructions:

- Arrange quinoa as the base in a bowl.

- Add steamed broccoli, bell peppers, shredded carrots, and avocado slices.

- Drizzle with a cooling tahini dressing.

3. Minty Lemonade Smoothie:

- Ingredients:

- Fresh mint leaves
- Cucumber, peeled and chopped

- Pineapple chunks

- Coconut water

- Juice of one lemon

- Ice cubes

- Instructions:

- Blend mint leaves, cucumber, pineapple chunks, coconut water, and lemon juice until smooth.

- Add ice cubes and blend again for a refreshing smoothie.

4. Coconut-Cilantro Chutney:

- Ingredients:

- Fresh cilantro (coriander), chopped

- Grated coconut

- Green chilies, chopped (adjust to taste)

- Roasted cumin seeds

- Yogurt

- Salt to taste

- Instructions:

- Blend cilantro, grated coconut, green chilies, roasted cumin seeds, yogurt, and salt until smooth.

- Serve as a cooling accompaniment to meals.

5. Stir-Fried Asparagus with Turmeric:

- Ingredients:

- Asparagus spears, trimmed
- Ghee
- Turmeric powder
- Cumin seeds
- Salt and pepper to taste

- Instructions:

- Heat ghee in a pan, add cumin seeds, and let them sizzle.

- Add asparagus spears, turmeric powder, salt, and pepper.

- Stir-fry until asparagus is tender but still crisp.

6. Berry and Mint Sorbet:

- Ingredients:

- Mixed berries (strawberries, blueberries, raspberries)
- Fresh mint leaves
- Honey or agave syrup (optional)
- Lemon juice

- Instructions:

- Blend mixed berries, fresh mint leaves, and lemon juice until smooth.

- Sweeten with honey or agave syrup if desired.

- Freeze the mixture in a shallow dish, stirring occasionally for a sorbet-like texture.

7. Cardamom Rose Lassi:

- Ingredients:

- Yogurt
- Rose water
- Cardamom powder
- Honey
- Ice cubes

- Instructions:

- Blend yogurt, a splash of rose water, cardamom powder, and honey until frothy.

- Pour over ice cubes for a fragrant and cooling lassi.

8. Grilled Eggplant and Tomato Salad:

- Ingredients:

- Sliced eggplant
- Cherry tomatoes, halved
- Fresh basil leaves
- Balsamic glaze
- Olive oil

- Salt and pepper to taste
- **Instructions:**
  - Grill eggplant slices until tender.
  - Toss grilled eggplant, cherry tomatoes, and fresh basil leaves in a bowl.
  - Drizzle with balsamic glaze and olive oil. Season with salt and pepper.

These joyful Pitta recipes celebrate the vibrant flavors of fresh, cooling ingredients while maintaining the principles of Ayurveda. Experiment with these recipes, adjusting them to your taste preferences, and enjoy the pleasure of nourishing both your body and spirit. Cooking with love and mindfulness adds an extra layer of joy to the dining experience, supporting the balance of Pitta dosha.

Breakfast Delights for Pitta Harmony

Breakfast is often considered the most important meal of the day, and for individuals with a predominant Pitta dosha, choosing morning delights that balance the intensity of this dosha is crucial. Incorporating cooling, nourishing, and easy-to-digest foods can set the tone for a harmonious day. Here are some delightful Pitta-friendly breakfast recipes that bring joy and balance to your morning routine:

1. Cooling Chia Seed Pudding:
  ### - Ingredients:
    - Chia seeds
    - Coconut milk or almond milk
    - Fresh berries (blueberries, raspberries)
    - Coconut flakes
    - Maple syrup or honey (optional)
  ### - Instructions:
    - Mix chia seeds with coconut or almond milk and let it sit in the refrigerator overnight.
    - In the morning, top with fresh berries, coconut flakes, and a drizzle of maple syrup or honey.

2. Pitta-Balancing Smoothie Bowl:
  ### - Ingredients:
    - Frozen mango chunks
    - Pineapple chunks

- Spinach leaves

- Coconut water

- Fresh mint leaves

- Chia seeds or flaxseeds (optional)

- Instructions:

- Blend frozen mango, pineapple, spinach, fresh mint, and coconut water until smooth.

- Pour into a bowl and top with chia seeds or flaxseeds for added texture.

3. Avocado Toast with Cucumber:**

- Ingredients:

- Whole-grain bread or gluten-free bread

- Ripe avocado

- Thinly sliced cucumber

- Lemon juice

- Fresh dill

- Salt and pepper to taste

- Instructions:

- Mash ripe avocado and spread it on toasted bread.

- Top with thinly sliced cucumber, a squeeze of lemon juice, fresh dill, salt, and pepper.

4. Quinoa Porridge with Berries:**

- Ingredients:

- Cooked quinoa

- Almond milk or coconut milk

- Mixed berries (strawberries, blueberries)

- Chopped nuts (almonds, walnuts)

- Cinnamon and cardamom

- Instructions:

- Heat cooked quinoa with almond or coconut milk.

- Top with mixed berries, chopped nuts, and a sprinkle of cinnamon and cardamom.

5. Minty Green Pancakes:

- Ingredients:

- Spinach leaves

- Fresh mint leaves

- Buckwheat flour or whole-grain flour

- Almond milk

- Baking powder

- Maple syrup or honey

- Instructions:

- Blend spinach, fresh mint, buckwheat flour, almond milk, and baking powder until smooth.

- Cook pancakes on a griddle and serve with a drizzle of maple syrup or honey.

6. Saffron Infused Overnight Oats:
- **Ingredients:**
  - Rolled oats
  - Almond milk or coconut milk
  - Saffron strands
  - Chopped dates or raisins
  - Sliced almonds or pistachios
- **Instructions:**
  - Infuse saffron strands in almond or coconut milk overnight.
  - Mix rolled oats with saffron-infused milk, chopped dates or raisins, and top with sliced almonds or pistachios.

7. Coconut Yogurt Parfait:
- **Ingredients:**
  - Coconut yogurt
  - Fresh mango chunks
  - Granola (choose a Pitta-friendly option)
  - Shredded coconut
- **Instructions:**

- Layer coconut yogurt with fresh mango chunks, granola, and shredded coconut in a parfait glass.

8. Turmeric Latte Oatmeal:
- **Ingredients:**
    - Rolled oats
    - Almond milk or coconut milk
    - Ground turmeric
    - Chopped nuts (cashews, almonds)
    - Honey or maple syrup
- **Instructions:**
    - Cook rolled oats with almond or coconut milk, stirring in ground turmeric.
    - Top with chopped nuts and a drizzle of honey or maple syrup.

These joyful Pitta recipes for breakfast not only cater to the specific needs of Pitta dosha but also infuse your morning with flavors and textures that bring joy and balance. Remember to adjust recipes based on your taste preferences and dietary needs. Cooking with love and mindfulness not only supports the balance of Pitta dosha but also enhances the overall enjoyment of your meals.

Lunchtime Elixirs for Energy and Balance

Lunch is a significant part of the day, providing an opportunity to refuel and nourish the body. For individuals with a predominant Pitta dosha, choosing lunchtime elixirs that incorporate cooling, soothing, and balancing ingredients is essential. These recipes not only support the unique needs of Pitta dosha but also bring joy and vitality to your midday meal. Here are some delightful Pitta-friendly lunchtime elixirs to infuse your afternoon with energy and balance:

1. Cucumber and Mint Gazpacho:
  - **Ingredients:**
    - Cucumbers, peeled and chopped
    - Tomatoes, chopped
    - Red bell pepper, chopped
    - Red onion, finely chopped

- Fresh mint leaves

- Garlic, minced

- Vegetable broth

- Olive oil

- Lemon juice

- Salt and pepper to taste

- Instructions:

- Blend cucumbers, tomatoes, red bell pepper, red onion, mint, and garlic with vegetable broth.

- Add olive oil, lemon juice, salt, and pepper.

- Chill in the refrigerator before serving.

2. Spinach and Fennel Salad with Citrus Vinaigrette:

- Ingredients:

- Fresh spinach leaves

- Sliced fennel

- Orange segments

- Grapefruit segments

- Toasted pine nuts

- Olive oil

- Balsamic vinegar

- Dijon mustard

- Honey

- Salt and pepper to taste

- Instructions:

- Toss spinach, fennel, orange segments, grapefruit segments, and toasted pine nuts in a bowl.

- Whisk together olive oil, balsamic vinegar, Dijon mustard, honey, salt, and pepper to create a citrus vinaigrette.

3. Pitta-Pacifying Quinoa Salad:

- Ingredients:
- Cooked quinoa
- Sliced cucumber
- Cherry tomatoes, halved
- Kalamata olives, pitted and sliced
- Feta cheese, crumbled
- Fresh oregano leaves
- Olive oil
- Lemon juice
- Salt and pepper to taste

- Instructions:

- Combine quinoa, cucumber, cherry tomatoes, olives, feta cheese, and fresh oregano in a bowl.

- Drizzle with olive oil and lemon juice. Season with salt and pepper.

4. Coconut-Cilantro Chickpea Curry:
- Ingredients:
- Chickpeas, cooked
- Coconut milk
- Fresh cilantro (coriander), chopped
- Tomatoes, diced
- Onion, finely chopped
- Garlic, minced
- Ginger, grated
- Turmeric powder
- Cumin powder
- Coriander powder
- Garam masala
- Salt and pepper to taste

- Instructions:
- In a pan, sauté onion, garlic, and ginger until fragrant.
- Add tomatoes, coconut milk, turmeric, cumin, coriander, garam masala, salt, and pepper.
- Stir in cooked chickpeas and simmer until flavors meld. Garnish with fresh cilantro.

5. Minty Zucchini Noodles with Pesto:

  - **Ingredients:**
    - Zucchini, spiralized into noodles
    - Fresh mint leaves
    - Pine nuts
    - Parmesan cheese (optional)
    - Garlic, minced
    - Olive oil
    - Lemon juice
    - Salt and pepper to taste

  - **Instructions:**

    - In a blender, combine fresh mint, pine nuts, Parmesan (if using), garlic, olive oil, lemon juice, salt, and pepper to create a minty pesto.

    - Toss zucchini noodles with the minty pesto.

6. Cooling Lentil and Mint Soup:

  - **Ingredients:**
    - Lentils, rinsed
    - Vegetable broth
    - Carrots, diced
    - Celery, diced
    - Fresh mint leaves

- Cumin seeds

- Coriander powder

- Lemon zest

- Olive oil

- Salt and pepper to taste

- Instructions:

- In a pot, sauté cumin seeds in olive oil until fragrant.

- Add lentils, vegetable broth, carrots, celery, fresh mint, coriander powder, lemon zest, salt, and pepper.

- Simmer until lentils are cooked.

7. Turmeric-Ginger Grilled Salmon:

- Ingredients:

- Salmon fillets

- Turmeric powder

- Ginger, grated

- Garlic, minced

- Lemon juice

- Olive oil

- Fresh cilantro (coriander), chopped

- Salt and pepper to taste

- Instructions:

- Mix turmeric, ginger, garlic, lemon juice, olive oil, cilantro, salt, and pepper to create a marinade.

- Coat salmon fillets with the marinade and grill until cooked.

8. Cooling Avocado and Cucumber Wraps:
- **Ingredients:**
  - Collard green leaves
  - Avocado slices
  - Sliced cucumber
  - Shredded carrots
  - Hummus
  - Alfalfa sprouts
  - Lemon wedges
  - Salt and pepper to taste
- **Instructions:**

- Lay collard green leaves flat and fill with avocado slices, cucumber, shredded carrots, hummus, and alfalfa sprouts.

- Sprinkle with salt and pepper, squeeze lemon juice, and wrap into a delightful roll.

These lunchtime elixirs for Pitta dosha not only offer cooling and balancing properties but also bring joy and satisfaction to your midday meals. Feel free to experiment with these recipes, adjusting ingredients based on your preferences and dietary needs. Cooking with love and intention adds an extra layer of joy and nourishment to your lunchtime experience.

Dinner Delicacies for Restful Pitta Nights

Dinner is a time to unwind and nourish the body, preparing it for a restful night. For individuals with a predominant Pitta dosha, choosing dinner delicacies that incorporate calming, grounding, and easily digestible ingredients is crucial. These recipes not only align with the principles of Ayurveda to balance Pitta dosha but also bring joy and satisfaction to your evening meals. Here are some delightful Pitta-friendly dinner recipes to ensure restful nights and harmonious well-being:

1. Coconut-Curried Sweet Potato Soup:
  - **Ingredients:**

- Sweet potatoes, peeled and diced
- Coconut milk
- Vegetable broth
- Curry powder
- Turmeric powder
- Ginger, grated
- Garlic, minced
- Cilantro (coriander), chopped
- Coconut oil
- Salt and pepper to taste

- **Instructions:**

- In a pot, sauté ginger and garlic in coconut oil.

- Add sweet potatoes, curry powder, turmeric, vegetable broth, and coconut milk.

- Simmer until sweet potatoes are tender. Garnish with chopped cilantro.

2. Cooling Cauliflower and Mint Pilaf:

- **Ingredients:**
  - Cauliflower rice
  - Fresh mint leaves, chopped
  - Peas
  - Sliced almonds
  - Ghee

- Cumin seeds

- Cardamom powder

- Turmeric powder

- Salt and pepper to taste

- Instructions:

- In a pan, sauté cumin seeds in ghee until they sizzle.

- Add cauliflower rice, peas, sliced almonds, cardamom, turmeric, salt, and pepper.

- Stir in fresh mint before serving.

3. Grilled Portobello Mushrooms with Herbed Quinoa:

- Ingredients:

- Portobello mushrooms, cleaned and stems removed

- Quinoa, cooked

- Fresh parsley, chopped

- Lemon zest

- Garlic, minced

- Olive oil

- Balsamic vinegar

- Salt and pepper to taste

- Instructions:

- Marinate portobello mushrooms in a mixture of olive oil, balsamic vinegar, garlic, salt, and pepper.

- Grill until tender. Serve over herbed quinoa garnished with fresh parsley and lemon zest.

4. Pitta-Soothing Dal with Spinach:

- Ingredients:

- Yellow lentils (moong dal), rinsed
- Spinach, chopped
- Ghee
- Cumin seeds
- Turmeric powder
- Coriander powder
- Asafoetida (hing)
- Ginger, grated
- Garlic, minced
- Tomatoes, diced
- Fresh cilantro (coriander), chopped
- Lemon wedges
- Salt and pepper to taste

- Instructions:

- In a pot, sauté cumin seeds in ghee until they sizzle.

- Add asafoetida, ginger, garlic, turmeric, coriander, lentils, and tomatoes.

- Cook until lentils are soft. Stir in chopped spinach and cook until wilted.

- Garnish with fresh cilantro and serve with a squeeze of lemon.

5. Baked Lemon Herb Salmon:

- **Ingredients:**
  - Salmon fillets
  - Fresh dill, chopped
  - Fresh parsley, chopped
  - Lemon zest
  - Garlic, minced
  - Olive oil
  - Lemon slices
  - Salt and pepper to taste

- **Instructions:**

- Preheat the oven. Mix dill, parsley, lemon zest, minced garlic, olive oil, salt, and pepper to create a marinade.

- Coat salmon fillets with the marinade and bake until cooked.

- Garnish with lemon slices before serving.

6. Zesty Chickpea and Cucumber Salad:

- Ingredients:

- Chickpeas, cooked
- Cucumber, diced
- Red onion, finely chopped
- Cherry tomatoes, halved
- Feta cheese, crumbled
- Kalamata olives, pitted and sliced
- Olive oil
- Lemon juice
- Fresh oregano leaves
- Salt and pepper to taste

- Instructions:

- Combine chickpeas, cucumber, red onion, cherry tomatoes, feta cheese, and olives in a bowl.

- Drizzle with olive oil and lemon juice. Season with fresh oregano, salt, and pepper.

7. Cooling Raita with Cumin and Mint:

- Ingredients:

- Yogurt
- Cucumber, grated
- Fresh mint leaves, chopped

- Cumin powder

- Salt to taste

- Instructions:

- Mix yogurt, grated cucumber, chopped mint, cumin powder, and salt to create a refreshing raita.

- Serve as a side dish to complement your main course.

8. Lentil and Vegetable Stuffed Bell Peppers:

- Ingredients:

- Bell peppers, halved

- Lentils, cooked

- Mixed vegetables (carrots, peas, corn)

- Onion, finely chopped

- Garlic, minced

- Tomato sauce

- Italian herbs (oregano, basil)

- Olive oil

- Salt and pepper to taste

- Instructions:

- Sauté onion and garlic in olive oil until translucent.

- Mix cooked lentils, mixed vegetables, tomato sauce, Italian herbs, salt, and pepper.

- Stuff bell peppers with the lentil and vegetable mixture and bake until peppers are tender.

These dinner delicacies for Pitta dosha not only promote restful nights but also infuse your evening with flavors that bring joy and satisfaction. Adjust the recipes to suit your taste preferences and dietary needs, and enjoy the pleasure of nourishing your body and soul. Cooking with mindfulness and intention adds an extra layer of joy to your dinner experience, supporting the balance of Pitta dosha.

Chapter 5: Lifestyle Practices for Pitta Harmony

Ayurveda, the ancient system of holistic healing, places a strong emphasis on maintaining balance among the doshas for overall well-being. For individuals with a predominant Pitta dosha, adopting lifestyle practices that align with Pitta's qualities can help promote harmony, calmness, and vitality. Here are some lifestyle practices tailored to support Pitta dosha balance:

1. Mindful Morning Routine:
  - **Early Rising:** Wake up early, ideally before sunrise, to align with the natural rhythm of the day.
  - **Hydration:** Start your day with a glass of room temperature water to rehydrate and stimulate the digestive system.
  - **Gentle Exercise:** Engage in gentle exercises like yoga or walking to invigorate the body without overexertion.

2. Cooling Self-Care Rituals:

- **Cooling Showers:** Opt for cool or lukewarm showers to soothe the skin and cool the body.

- **Aromatherapy:** Use calming essential oils such as lavender, mint, or rose in diffusers or during self-massage.

3. Balanced Diet:

- **Pitta-Pacifying Foods:** Emphasize a diet rich in cooling and hydrating foods, including leafy greens, sweet fruits, and whole grains.

- **Regular Meals:** Eat regular, well-balanced meals at consistent times to support stable blood sugar levels.

4. Mindful Eating:

- **Chew Thoroughly:** Practice mindful eating by chewing your food thoroughly to aid digestion and avoid overeating.

- **Enjoy Cooling Teas:** Sip on herbal teas like mint, coriander, or fennel throughout the day to balance internal heat.

5. Strategic Workouts:

- **Yoga and Tai Chi:** Engage in yoga or Tai Chi to cultivate mindfulness, flexibility, and balance.

- **Avoid Excessive Heat:** Choose workouts that avoid overheating, and practice in a cool environment.

6. Stress Management:

- **Mind-Body Practices:** Incorporate stress-reducing practices such as meditation, deep breathing, or mindfulness to calm the mind.

- **Time in Nature:** Spend time in nature to ground yourself and connect with the calming energy of the outdoors.

7. Regular Breaks:

- **Balanced Work Routine:** Incorporate breaks during work to prevent overexertion and maintain focus.

- **Short Walks:** Take short walks to clear your mind and provide a refreshing break.

8. Cultivate Creativity:

- **Artistic Pursuits:** Engage in creative activities such as painting, writing, or music to channel your energy into expressive outlets.

- **Mindful Hobbies:** Pursue hobbies that bring joy and relaxation without triggering excessive intensity.

9. Cooling Sleep Environment:

- **Comfortable Bedding:** Invest in comfortable, breathable bedding to promote restful sleep.

- **Cooling Colors:** Choose cool and calming colors for your bedroom to create a restful atmosphere.

10. Pace Yourself:

- **Avoid Overcommitting:** Be mindful of your schedule and avoid overcommitting to prevent burnout.

- **Prioritize Rest:** Ensure you get enough restorative sleep each night to recharge your energy.

11. Cultivate Compassion:

- **Practice Self-Compassion:** Be kind to yourself and avoid self-criticism. Cultivate self-compassion through positive affirmations.

- **Express Gratitude:** Regularly express gratitude to shift focus away from stressors and enhance a positive mindset.

12. Embrace Routine and Structure:

- **Consistent Bedtime:** Aim for a consistent bedtime to regulate your sleep-wake cycle.

- **Structured Days:** Establish a daily routine to provide a sense of structure and stability.

13. Cooling Skincare:

- **Gentle Cleansers:** Use gentle, cooling skincare products to soothe sensitive skin.

- **Sun Protection:** Prioritize sun protection with natural, non-comedogenic sunscreens to prevent skin irritation.

14. **Limit Stimulants:

- **Caffeine Moderation:** Consume caffeine in moderation and be mindful of its stimulating effects.

- **Avoid Excessive Spices:** Limit the use of hot and spicy foods that can exacerbate internal heat.

15. Digital Detox:

- **Screen Time Awareness:** Be mindful of screen time and take breaks to reduce eye strain.
- **Quiet Time:** Create periods of quiet time without electronic devices to promote mental calmness.

Incorporating these lifestyle practices into your daily routine can help individuals with a predominant Pitta dosha maintain balance, enhance well-being, and foster a harmonious connection with mind, body, and spirit. However, it's essential to remember that Ayurveda is highly individualized, and consulting with an Ayurvedic practitioner can provide personalized guidance based on your unique constitution and health goals.

Mindful Eating and Digestive Health

In Ayurveda, mindful eating is a fundamental aspect of promoting overall well-being, especially for individuals with a predominant Pitta dosha. Pitta, characterized by fire and water elements, governs digestion, and maintaining its balance is crucial for optimal health. Here are mindful eating and digestive health practices tailored to support Pitta dosha harmony:

1. Eat at Regular Intervals:
  - **Establish a Routine:** Eat meals at consistent times each day to support the natural rhythm of your digestive system.
  - **Avoid Skipping Meals:** Pitta benefits from regular nourishment, and skipping meals can lead to imbalances.

2. Choose Pitta-Pacifying Foods:
  - **Cooling Foods:** Prioritize cooling and hydrating foods such as sweet fruits, leafy greens, and dairy in moderation.

- **Avoid Excessive Heat:** Minimize the consumption of overly spicy, hot, or fried foods that can exacerbate internal heat.

3. Mindful Food Choices:

- **Conscious Selection:** Be mindful of the quality and source of your food. Choose fresh, whole, and organic options when possible.

- **Variety and Moderation:** Include a variety of foods in your diet, and practice moderation to avoid overloading your digestive system.

4. Chew Thoroughly:

- **Slow and Steady:** Chew your food thoroughly and savor each bite. Eating slowly allows the digestive process to begin in the mouth.

- **Digestive Enzymes:** Chewing activates digestive enzymes in saliva, aiding the breakdown of food for easier absorption.

5. Mindful Mealtime Atmosphere:

- **Create a Calm Setting:** Eat in a peaceful environment with minimal distractions. Avoid stressful discussions or intense activities during meals.

- **Soft Lighting:** Opt for soft, calming lighting to create a soothing atmosphere.

6. Hydration Habits:

- **Sip Warm Water:** Drink warm water throughout the day to support digestion. Avoid ice-cold beverages, as they can dampen the digestive fire.
- **Herbal Teas:** Enjoy Pitta-pacifying herbal teas like mint, coriander, or fennel between meals.

7. Digestive Spices:

- **Cumin and Coriander:** Include digestive spices like cumin and coriander in your meals to enhance digestion and balance Pitta.
- **Mint:** Add fresh mint to meals or drinks for its cooling and digestive properties.

8. Prefer Fresh and Light Meals:

- **Seasonal Eating:** Embrace seasonal, fresh produce as they align with nature and support digestive harmony.

- **Light Dinners:** Choose lighter meals for dinner to avoid overloading your digestive system before bedtime.

9. Avoid Emotional Eating:

- **Mind-Body Connection:** Be aware of emotional triggers for eating. Practice mindfulness to differentiate between physical hunger and emotional cravings.

- **Choose Nourishment:** Prioritize nourishing your body over emotional satisfaction through food.

10. Gentle Exercise After Meals:

- **Post-Meal Walks:** Take a leisurely stroll after meals to aid digestion. Avoid intense workouts immediately after eating.

- **Gentle Yoga Poses:** Practice gentle yoga poses that focus on digestion, such as seated twists or forward bends.

11. Herbal Support for Digestion:

- **Triphala:** Consider incorporating triphala, an Ayurvedic herbal formulation, to support gentle cleansing and digestive health.

- **Ginger Tea:** Sip on ginger tea, known for its digestive properties, between meals.

12. Mindful Portion Control:

- **Listen to Hunger Cues:**** Pay attention to your body's hunger and fullness signals. Avoid overeating by tuning into your body's natural cues.

- **Quality Over Quantity:** Focus on the quality of your food rather than quantity. Choose nutrient-dense options for optimal nourishment.

13. Regular Detoxification:

- **Seasonal Cleansing:** Consider seasonal Ayurvedic cleansing practices to eliminate toxins and support digestive rejuvenation.

- **Fasting Mindfully:** If fasting, do so mindfully and choose methods that align with your constitution and health goals.

14. Manage Stress:

- **Stress Reduction Techniques:** Engage in stress-reducing activities such as meditation, deep breathing, or mindfulness to promote a calm and balanced mind.

- **Avoid Stressful Conversations:** Avoid engaging in stressful discussions during meals to allow for optimal digestion.

15. Reflect on Your Meals:

- **Gratitude Practice:** Cultivate a sense of gratitude for the food you consume. Reflect on the effort and energy that went into providing nourishment.

- **Digestive Journaling:** Consider keeping a journal to track your meals, notice how your body responds, and identify any patterns related to digestion.

Adopting these mindful eating and digestive health practices can help individuals with a predominant Pitta dosha maintain balance and support optimal well-being. It's essential to listen to your body, make adjustments based on personal needs, and seek guidance from an Ayurvedic practitioner for a more personalized approach to mindful living.

Daily Routines for Pitta Balance

Lifestyle practices play a crucial role in maintaining balance and harmony in the body, mind, and spirit, according to Ayurveda, the ancient system of holistic healing from India. In Ayurveda, individuals are classified into three doshas—Vata, Pitta, and Kapha—each representing a unique combination of elements. Pitta, composed of fire and water elements, governs metabolism, digestion, and transformation in the body.

For those with a predominant Pitta constitution or experiencing a Pitta imbalance, adopting specific lifestyle practices can help restore equilibrium. Here are some daily routines and practices to foster Pitta harmony:

1. **Early Rise and Shine:**
   Pitta is associated with the fire element, and the early morning hours are considered the time of day when this energy is most dominant. Wake up before sunrise to align with the natural rhythm of

the day. This will help you start your day with a sense of calm and freshness.

2. **Cooling Morning Routine:**
Begin your day with a refreshing splash of cool water on your face and eyes. Opt for a gentle, cooling skincare routine to pacify any excess heat in the skin. Aloe vera gel or rose water can be beneficial.

3. **Hydrate with Room Temperature Water:**
Pitta individuals should stay well-hydrated to balance their internal heat. Sip on room temperature water throughout the day, and consider adding a slice of cucumber or mint for an extra cooling effect.

4. **Mindful Breakfast:**
Favor a Pitta-pacifying breakfast that includes sweet, bitter, and astringent tastes. Opt for cooling foods like oatmeal, fresh fruits, and coconut. Avoid spicy or overly heating foods to prevent aggravating Pitta.

5. **Moderate Exercise:**

Engage in moderate, non-competitive exercises such as swimming, walking, or yoga. Pitta benefits from activities that promote a sense of calm and relaxation without overheating the body.

6. **Pitta-Pacifying Diet:**

Emphasize cooling and hydrating foods in your meals. Incorporate sweet, bitter, and astringent tastes while reducing pungent, sour, and salty foods. Include plenty of leafy greens, cucumbers, coconut, and sweet fruits.

7. **Take Regular Breaks:**

Pitta individuals tend to be driven and ambitious. However, it's essential to take breaks to prevent burnout. Schedule short breaks during work or study to cool down and relax your mind.

8. **Cooling Herbal Teas:**

Enjoy herbal teas that have cooling properties, such as mint, fennel, or chamomile. These teas can help balance Pitta and soothe the digestive system.

9. **Avoid Overheating:**

Pitta individuals should be cautious about excessive sun exposure, especially during the peak hours of the day. Use natural sun protection like hats and wear breathable fabrics to stay cool.

10. **Relaxing Evening Routine:**

Wind down in the evening with calming activities. A gentle stroll, meditation, or reading a soothing book can help transition into a restful night's sleep.

Remember, Ayurveda is a personalized science, and what works for one person may not be suitable for another. It's advisable to consult with an Ayurvedic practitioner to determine your unique constitution and imbalances for a more tailored approach to achieving Pitta harmony.

Yoga and Meditation for Pitta Well-Being

Yoga and meditation are powerful tools for promoting balance and harmony within the Pitta dosha. These practices not only help to calm the mind but also contribute to cooling the body and reducing excess heat associated with Pitta. Here are some specific yoga and meditation practices tailored for Pitta well-being:

Yoga for Pitta Harmony:

1. Gentle Asanas:

Choose yoga poses that are gentle, calming, and focus on flexibility rather than intensity. Include poses that open the chest and promote relaxation, such as child's pose, cobra pose, and gentle twists.

2. Cooling Pranayama:

Incorporate pranayama (breath control) practices that have a cooling effect on the body. Sheetali and Sheetkari pranayamas involve inhaling through the mouth with a curled tongue or through the teeth, respectively, creating a cooling sensation.

3. Moon Salutations:

Include Moon Salutations (Chandra Namaskar) in your practice. These sequences are designed to channel the calming, receptive energy of the moon, helping to balance the heat of Pitta.

4. Restorative Yoga:

Embrace restorative yoga poses that encourage relaxation and release tension. Supported poses with props, such as bolsters and blankets, can be particularly beneficial for calming Pitta energy.

5. Mindful Movement:

Practice yoga mindfully, paying attention to the sensations in your body. Avoid pushing yourself too hard or practicing in overly heated environments. Opt for cool, well-ventilated spaces.

Meditation for Pitta Well-Being:

1. Mindfulness Meditation:

Engage in mindfulness meditation to cultivate awareness and presence. Focus on the breath, observing each inhalation and exhalation. This practice can help calm the mind and reduce stress, a key factor in balancing Pitta.

2. Visualization:

Use visualization techniques to imagine cool, serene landscapes. Picture a calming blue ocean or a lush green forest to bring a sense of peace and tranquility, counteracting the heat of Pitta.

3. Loving-Kindness Meditation:

Practice loving-kindness meditation to cultivate feelings of compassion and warmth. Extend feelings of love and goodwill to yourself and others. This can help balance the intensity often associated with Pitta.

4. Chandra Bhedana (Left Nostril Breathing):

This specific pranayama involves breathing through the left nostril, associated with the moon and the cooling energy in the body. It can help balance Pitta and induce a sense of calm.

5. Body Scan Meditation:

Conduct a body scan meditation to release tension and heat from different parts of the body. Start from the toes and gradually move up to the head, consciously relaxing each area.

Remember, consistency is key when incorporating yoga and meditation into your routine for Pitta harmony. It's advisable to listen to your body and modify practices based on your energy levels and comfort. Additionally, consulting with a qualified yoga instructor or meditation guide can provide personalized guidance for your specific Pitta constitution and imbalances.

Chapter 6: Savoring the Joy of Pitta Balance

Savoring the joy of Pitta balance involves embracing a harmonious and mindful approach to life that nurtures the qualities of this dosha without allowing them to become excessive. Pitta individuals are often driven, ambitious, and focused, and achieving balance entails appreciating these attributes while avoiding overexertion and stress. Here are some ways to savor the joy of Pitta balance:

1. Celebrate Achievements with Moderation:

Pitta individuals are naturally ambitious and enjoy setting and achieving goals. While accomplishments are worthy of celebration, it's crucial to do so with moderation. Avoid excessive self-criticism or an all-or-nothing mentality, and take the time to appreciate your achievements mindfully.

2. Cultivate Gratitude:

Foster a sense of gratitude for the positive aspects of your life. Keep a gratitude journal to reflect on the things you are thankful for. Gratitude can help shift focus from perfectionism to acknowledging and appreciating the joy in everyday moments.

3. Enjoy Healthy Competition:

Pitta individuals thrive in competitive environments, but it's essential to keep it healthy and enjoyable. Choose activities that challenge and motivate you without fostering stress or aggression. Friendly competition can add excitement and joy to your pursuits.

4. Savor Culinary Delights Mindfully:

Pitta individuals often have a keen appreciation for good food. Enjoy the pleasures of the dining experience by savoring each bite mindfully. Opt for cooling and nourishing foods that support Pitta balance, and take time to appreciate the flavors and textures.

5. Engage in Creative Pursuits:

Pitta individuals have a creative spark that thrives when expressed. Channel your creativity into activities that bring joy, whether it's painting, writing, or playing a musical instrument. This allows you to enjoy the process without being solely focused on the end result.

6. Balanced Social Interactions:

Socialize with a diverse group of people and engage in activities that bring joy and connection. Pitta individuals may benefit from balancing their driven nature with the lightheartedness of social interactions. Choose social activities that are fun and foster a sense of camaraderie.

7. Cooling Leisure Activities:

Incorporate leisure activities that have a cooling effect on the body and mind. Consider activities such as swimming, spending time in nature, or enjoying a leisurely stroll in the evening. These activities help to counteract the natural heat associated with Pitta.

8. Mindful Rest and Relaxation:

Embrace rest and relaxation as an integral part of your routine. Pitta individuals may be prone to overworking, so taking time for restorative practices, such as meditation, gentle yoga, or simply unwinding with a good book, is essential for maintaining balance and joy.

9. Practice Mindful Breathing:

Incorporate mindful breathing exercises to stay present and centered. Deep, slow breaths can help alleviate stress and prevent Pitta from becoming overly dominant. This practice fosters a sense of calm and joy in the midst of daily challenges.

10. Prioritize Playfulness:

Infuse an element of playfulness into your life. Engage in activities that bring out your inner child, whether it's playing a sport, dancing, or enjoying a game night with friends and family. Playfulness adds a joyful dimension to the Pitta temperament.

In essence, savoring the joy of Pitta balance involves appreciating your unique qualities while making conscious choices to prevent them from tipping into excess. By incorporating mindfulness, gratitude, and a balanced approach to life, you can embrace the vitality and enthusiasm that Pitta brings without compromising your well-being.

Building Sustainable Ayurvedic Habits

Savoring the joy of Pitta balance goes hand-in-hand with building sustainable Ayurvedic habits. Ayurveda, the ancient system of holistic healing from India, emphasizes the importance of aligning daily routines and habits with one's unique dosha constitution. For those with a predominant Pitta dosha or experiencing Pitta imbalances, incorporating sustainable Ayurvedic habits can bring about lasting well-being. Here are some practices to help build and savor the joy of Pitta balance:

1. Rise with the Sun:

Establish a consistent wake-up routine that aligns with the natural rhythm of the day. Pitta individuals benefit from waking up early, ideally before sunrise, to harness the cool, calm energy of the early morning.

2. Mindful Morning Rituals:

Create a morning routine that promotes mindfulness and sets a positive tone for the day. Incorporate practices like tongue scraping, oil pulling, and a refreshing cool water face splash to cleanse and invigorate the senses.

3. Nourishing Breakfast:

Begin your day with a nourishing breakfast that includes cooling and sweet tastes. Opt for foods such as oatmeal, fresh fruits, and a touch of ghee to support balanced energy throughout the morning.

4. Pitta-Pacifying Diet:

Adopt a Pitta-pacifying diet by favoring foods that are sweet, bitter, and astringent. Include cooling foods like leafy greens, cucumbers, coconut, and grains like barley and basmati rice. Eat mindfully, savoring each bite and paying attention to your body's signals.

5. Hydrate Wisely:

Stay well-hydrated by sipping room temperature water throughout the day. Infuse your water with slices of cucumber, mint, or a splash of lime for added refreshing benefits. Avoid excessive consumption of iced or extremely cold beverages.

6. Cooling Herbal Teas:

Incorporate Ayurvedic herbs and teas known for their cooling properties. Peppermint, fennel, and chamomile teas can help pacify Pitta and promote a sense of calm.

7. Balanced Work and Rest:

Structure your workday to include breaks and moments of relaxation. Pitta individuals may be prone to overworking, so establishing a healthy work-rest balance is crucial for sustainable well-being.

8. Mindful Movement:

Engage in moderate exercise that supports Pitta balance without causing excessive heat. Practices like swimming, walking, or gentle yoga are ideal for maintaining physical health without overstimulating the system.

9. Creative Expression:

Channel your creative energy into activities that bring joy and fulfillment. Whether it's writing, painting, or playing an instrument, expressing yourself creatively helps to balance Pitta's intense drive with the joy of creation.

10. Mindful Evening Routine:

Wind down your day with a calming evening routine. Avoid stimulating activities close to bedtime and opt for practices like meditation, gentle yoga, or reading a calming book to prepare your mind and body for restful sleep.

11. Prioritize Quality Sleep:

Establish a consistent sleep schedule and create a sleep-friendly environment. Pitta individuals benefit from quality sleep to allow the body to cool down and rejuvenate. Ensure your bedroom is cool, dark, and conducive to rest.

12. Reflection and Gratitude:

Take time for self-reflection and express gratitude for the positive aspects of your day. This practice helps to cultivate a positive mindset and fosters a sense of joy in daily living.

Building sustainable Ayurvedic habits for Pitta balance involves creating a lifestyle that is nourishing, mindful, and aligned with the principles of Ayurveda. By embracing these practices consistently, individuals can savor the joy of Pitta balance and experience lasting well-being in their physical, mental, and emotional realms.

Nurturing Pitta Dosha for Long-Term Health

Savoring the joy of Pitta balance involves nurturing the Pitta dosha for long-term health and well-being. Pitta, associated with the elements of fire and water, governs digestion, metabolism, and transformation in the body. To sustain a harmonious Pitta balance, it's essential to adopt nurturing practices that cool and soothe this dosha. Here are key elements to consider in nurturing the Pitta dosha for long-term health:

1. Mindful Nutrition:

Foster a mindful and nourishing approach to nutrition. Choose cooling, Pitta-pacifying foods that include sweet, bitter, and astringent tastes. Incorporate plenty of fresh fruits, vegetables, whole grains, and lean proteins into your diet while minimizing spicy, oily, and acidic foods.

2. Pitta-Soothing Herbs:

Integrate Ayurvedic herbs known for their Pitta-soothing properties into your routine. Aloe vera, mint, coriander, and fennel can be beneficial in calming excess Pitta. Consider consulting with an Ayurvedic practitioner to find the right herbs for your individual needs.

3. Regular Exercise with Awareness:

Engage in regular, moderate exercise that promotes balance without overheating the body. Pitta individuals may enjoy activities like swimming, hiking, or yoga. Pay attention to your body's signals and avoid excessive intensity or overheating during workouts.

4. Balanced Lifestyle:

Strive for a balanced lifestyle that includes a mix of work, rest, and play. Pitta individuals often have a strong work ethic, but it's crucial to incorporate periods of relaxation and recreation to prevent burnout and maintain equilibrium.

5. Manage Stress:

Pitta individuals are prone to stress due to their ambitious nature. Practice stress-management techniques such as meditation, deep breathing, and mindfulness to foster emotional well-being. Create a routine that includes moments of calm and reflection.

6. Cooling Therapies:

Explore cooling therapies to balance the internal heat associated with Pitta. Abhyanga, or self-massage with coconut or sunflower oil, can have a cooling effect on the body. Additionally, consider occasional massages with cooling oils like coconut or sandalwood.

7. Hydration:

Stay well-hydrated to support the body's natural detoxification processes. Sip on room temperature water throughout the day and consider herbal teas with cooling properties. Avoid excessive consumption of caffeinated or sugary beverages.

8. Pitta-Friendly Skincare:

Choose skincare products that are gentle, hydrating, and soothing. Look for products with natural ingredients like aloe vera, cucumber, and rose, which help to cool and calm the skin. Protect your skin from excessive sun exposure with a natural sunscreen.

9. Mindful Breathing:

Practice mindful breathing exercises to bring a sense of calm to the mind and body. Sheetali and Sheetkari pranayamas, which involve cooling the breath, can be particularly beneficial for balancing Pitta. Incorporate these practices into your daily routine.

10. Create a Cool Sleep Environment:

Prioritize quality sleep by creating a cool and comfortable sleep environment. Ensure your bedroom is well-ventilated, and use lightweight, breathable bedding. Going to bed before 10 p.m. aligns with Pitta's natural rhythm.

11. Seasonal Awareness:

Adjust your lifestyle and habits according to the seasons. Pitta tends to be more pronounced in the summer, so pay extra attention to staying cool during hot weather. Adjust your diet, exercise routine, and self-care practices accordingly.

12. Regular Detoxification:

Support the body's detoxification processes through occasional cleansing practices. This can include gentle detoxifying diets, fasting, or Ayurvedic therapies like Panchakarma. Consult with an Ayurvedic practitioner for personalized guidance.

Savoring the joy of Pitta balance is a journey of self-care and mindful living. By incorporating these nurturing practices into your daily life, you can support the Pitta dosha for long-term health and experience the joy that comes with a balanced, vibrant, and harmonious existence.

Celebrating Wellness: Your Journey to Joy

"Savoring the Joy of Pitta Balance: Celebrating Wellness - Your Journey to Joy" encapsulates the essence of embracing a holistic approach to well-being while honoring the unique qualities of the Pitta dosha. Celebrating wellness is not merely a destination but an ongoing journey that involves cultivating joy in every aspect of life. Here's a guide to savoring the joy of Pitta balance and celebrating your journey to wellness:

1. Mindful Self-Discovery:

Embark on a journey of self-discovery to understand your unique constitution and the tendencies of your Pitta dosha. This awareness lays the foundation for making informed choices that align with your individual needs and promotes long-term well-being.

2. Gratitude as a Daily Practice:

Cultivate a daily practice of gratitude to appreciate the abundance in your life. Reflect on the positive aspects, acknowledging the joy found in even the smallest moments. Gratitude serves as a powerful tool in creating a positive mindset and fostering a sense of contentment.

3. Joyful Movement and Exercise:

Infuse joy into your physical activities. Whether it's dancing, practicing yoga, or engaging in a sport, choose activities that bring pleasure and vitality. The joy derived from movement not only enhances physical health but also positively impacts mental and emotional well-being.

4. Nourishing Relationships:

Prioritize relationships that uplift and support your well-being. Nurture connections with family and friends who bring joy and positive energy into your life. Building strong, supportive relationships contributes significantly to a sense of fulfillment and happiness.

5. Mindful Eating for Pleasure and Health:

Approach eating as a joyful experience. Savor the flavors, textures, and aromas of your meals. Choose foods that nourish and pacify Pitta while bringing delight to your palate. Mindful eating enhances the digestive process and fosters a deeper connection with your body.

6. Creative Expression as a Source of Joy:

Embrace your creative instincts and express yourself through art, writing, music, or any other form of creative expression. Engaging in activities that tap into your creative reservoir not only brings joy but also serves as a cathartic outlet for emotions.

7. Rest and Rejuvenation:

Prioritize rest and rejuvenation as essential components of your wellness journey. Allow yourself moments of calm and relaxation, whether through meditation, deep breathing, or simply taking a leisurely stroll. Adequate rest ensures sustained vitality and joy.

8. Balancing Work and Play:

Strike a harmonious balance between your work and leisure. While productivity is essential, integrating moments of play and recreation into your routine is equally vital for a joyous and well-rounded life. Recognize the value of downtime to recharge and replenish.

9. Connection with Nature:

Immerse yourself in nature to experience its calming and grounding effects. Whether it's a stroll in the park, a hike in the mountains, or simply basking in the sunlight, connecting with nature fosters a sense of joy and awe, helping to balance Pitta's intensity.

10. Reflect and Adjust:

Regularly reflect on your wellness journey and make adjustments as needed. Celebrate your successes, learn from challenges, and fine-tune your lifestyle practices. The joy of balance comes from an adaptive and evolving approach to well-being.

11. Mindful Breathing for Inner Calm:

Integrate mindful breathing practices into your daily routine. Whether it's pranayama exercises or simply taking a few moments to focus on your breath, mindful breathing serves as an anchor for inner calm and joy.

12. Celebrate Milestones:

Acknowledge and celebrate your wellness milestones. Whether it's achieving a fitness goal, adopting a new healthy habit, or simply maintaining balance, take the time to appreciate and celebrate the steps you've taken on your journey to joy.

In savoring the joy of Pitta balance, it's essential to approach wellness holistically, considering the interconnectedness of the body, mind, and spirit. Celebrating your journey to joy involves embracing a mindful and joyous approach to every facet of life, recognizing that true well-being is a continuous and evolving celebration.

Conclusion

This journey through the world of Ayurveda with a focus on a beginner's cookbook, we've explored the rich tapestry of this ancient holistic healing system. Ayurveda, with its emphasis on balance, individualized wellness, and harmony with nature, extends its wisdom to the realm of nourishment through the Ayurveda Cookbook for Beginners.

This cookbook serves as a gateway, inviting individuals to embark on a culinary adventure that aligns with the principles of Ayurveda. By understanding one's unique constitution or dosha and incorporating the six tastes into daily meals, the cookbook empowers readers to foster balance and well-being through mindful and intentional eating.

The recipes provided offer a harmonious blend of flavors, textures, and nutritional elements, showcasing the versatility of Ayurvedic cooking. From comforting stews to vibrant salads, each dish is thoughtfully crafted to bring not only sustenance but also a sense of alignment with the body's natural rhythms.

Moreover, the Ayurveda Cookbook for Beginners extends beyond the kitchen, encouraging a holistic approach to health. It reinforces the importance of mindful eating, considering the source and quality of ingredients, as well as the connection between food and overall well-being.

As we close this culinary exploration, it's worth noting that Ayurveda is not merely a set of guidelines but a way of life—a philosophy that encourages individuals to attune themselves to the cyclical nature of existence, finding balance amidst life's fluctuations. By embracing Ayurvedic principles in the kitchen, we can cultivate not only physical health but also a deeper connection to the world around us.

In essence, the Ayurveda Cookbook for Beginners serves as a compass on the journey toward mindful, nourishing, and joyous living. It invites individuals to savor the flavors of balance, harness the healing potential of food, and embark on a transformative path toward holistic well-being. May this culinary odyssey be the beginning of a lifelong exploration into the wisdom of Ayurveda, bringing health, harmony, and joy to all who embark on this enriching journey.